LITTLE BOOK OF
KETO

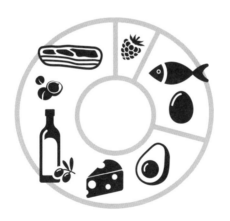

Taylor Spencer

THE LITTLE BOOK OF KETO

Text by Stephanie Parent

An Hachette UK Company
www.hachette.co.uk

Vie Books, an imprint of Summersdale Publishers Ltd
Part of Octopus Publishing Group Limited
Carmelite House
50 Victoria Embankment
LONDON
EC4Y 0DZ
UK

www.summersdale.com

Printed and bound in the UK

ISBN: 978-1-80007-680-8

Substantial discounts on bulk quantities of Summersdale books are available to corporations, professional associations and other organizations. For details contact general enquiries: telephone: +44 (0) 1243 771107 or email: enquiries@summersdale.com.

Contents

INTRODUCTION: SO YOU WANT TO KNOW MORE?   5

WHAT KETO MEANS: A BRIEF Q&A   6

RECIPES

    BREAKFAST   31
    LUNCH   48
    DINNER AND SIDES   65
    DESSERTS AND SNACKS   97

MEAL PLANNERS   117

THE DOs AND DON'Ts OF KETO   123

CONCLUSION   127

DISCLAIMER

Neither the author nor the publisher can be held responsible for any injury, loss or claim arising out of the use, or misuse, of the suggestions made herein. Always consult your doctor before trying any new diet if you have a medical or health condition, or are worried about any of the side effects. The keto diet is not safe for anyone with kidney, gallbladder, pancreas or thyroid disease.

INTRODUCTION:
SO YOU WANT TO KNOW MORE?

Welcome to *The Little Book of Keto*. Perhaps you've picked up this book as a complete newcomer to the ketogenic diet; perhaps you've heard about the health benefits of keto, or you have acquaintances who've lost weight or lowered their blood pressure after adopting a keto diet. Whatever your experience, this book will offer clear, concise explanations of how keto works, how it promotes health and how to adopt and stick to a keto diet yourself. You'll find plenty of easy, delicious and nutritious keto recipes for every meal of the day, along with meal plans and dos and don'ts to help you along your keto journey.

WHAT KETO MEANS: A BRIEF Q&A

THIS CHAPTER ANSWERS THE MOST
COMMON QUESTIONS ABOUT KETO – FROM
HOW THE DIET WORKS, TO WHAT YOU
CAN AND CAN'T EAT, WHAT BENEFITS
KETO OFFERS AND HOW TO STAY SAFE
WHILE FOLLOWING A KETO DIET. BY THE
END OF THIS CHAPTER, YOU'LL HAVE
THE INFORMATION YOU NEED TO DECIDE
WHETHER KETO'S THE RIGHT APPROACH
FOR YOU. ONCE YOU'RE READY TO TRY
KETO, YOU'LL FIND PLENTY OF
TIPS HERE TO PLAN AND FOLLOW
YOUR PERSONAL KETO DIET.

WHAT IS KETO?

"Keto" is shorthand for a ketogenic diet, a way of eating that brings about a state of ketosis in the body. During ketosis, the body uses fat rather than carbohydrates as its primary energy source. A ketogenic diet consists mainly of fat, along with a moderate amount of protein and as little as 5 to 10 per cent carbohydrates. By limiting carbohydrates, which usually fuel our brain and muscles, the keto diet forces the body to break down fat for energy instead. As the body burns off stored fat, weight loss and other health benefits can occur.

HOW DO YOU EAT KETO?

Following a ketogenic diet doesn't just mean limiting carbs – the diet requires a daily balance of 70 to 80 per cent calories from fat, 15 to 25 per cent from protein and the remainder from carbohydrates. In addition, keto completely eliminates carbohydrate-dense foods, such as grains, starchy vegetables, high-sugar fruits and simple sugars. Instead, the diet's carbohydrates come from low-carb vegetables and low-sugar fruits. Keeping the body's supply of carbs to a minimum ensures that the body can't use glucose as fuel. Without glucose, the body will turn to fat to power essential processes – a phenomenon we'll explore in depth in the next few pages.

HOW DOES IT WORK?

The keto diet works by starving your body of glucose – i.e. the human body's most basic energy source. During the digestive process, all carbohydrates – from whole grains to bread, pasta to fruit – break down into simple sugars called glucose. When consuming a carbohydrate-rich diet, the human body uses glucose to make adenosine triphosphate (ATP), a cellular fuel that helps muscles contract and nerve impulses to spread throughout the body. In short, ATP powers human movement and thought.

Without glucose, your body needs another way to synthesize ATP and keep cells functioning, so it turns to fat molecules. The body derives energy from fat through a process called ketosis.

WHAT DOES IT MEAN TO BE IN KETOSIS?

Ketosis is a metabolic state in which the body has exhausted its carbohydrate stores and must break down fats to fuel cells. During ketosis, the liver accesses stored or dietary fat and converts fatty acids into ketone bodies. These ketones are released from the liver into the bloodstream and travel to cells throughout the body, where they take over processes otherwise powered by glucose – producing ATP and driving cell function. The body reaches ketosis when ketones occur at a level of 0.5 to 3 millimoles per litre in the blood.

The body can enter ketosis during starvation, fasting or prolonged exercise – any state in which the glucose supply has been used up. The low-carb keto diet is a way to deliberately induce ketosis. Most people reach ketosis within two to four days of following a strict ketogenic diet, although the process can take up to ten days.

WHAT CAN YOU EAT?

In a keto diet, approximately three-quarters of daily calories come from fat. To optimize health while in ketosis, focus on heart-healthy fats: olive, coconut and avocado oils, fatty fish, avocados, nuts and seeds. Add saturated fats from eggs, beef, pork and high-fat dairy (butter, cream, yoghurt and cheese) only in moderation. Avoid lower-fat dairy like milk and low-fat yoghurt, which contain a higher percentage of sugar.

Protein from meat, poultry, fish, high-fat dairy, nuts and eggs should make up 15 to 25 per cent of daily food intake, with the rest coming from carbohydrates. Prioritize low-sugar carbs, such as leafy green and cruciferous vegetables (kale, cauliflower, broccoli, etc.), tomatoes, mushrooms, summer squash and berries. Low-carb almond and coconut flours are keto-friendly, and can be used to make bread, muffins and more.

Herbs and spices, vinegar and mustard can add savoury flavour to keto meals, while stevia is a substitute for sugar without adding carbs.

WHAT CAN'T YOU EAT?

Foods high in complex carbohydrates and/or simple sugars must be avoided to stay in ketosis. While following a keto diet, eliminate grains including bread, cereals, pasta, rice, tortillas, oats, quinoa, bulgur, barley and corn- or flour-based chips and crackers. Don't eat starchy, high-carb vegetables like potatoes, sweet potatoes, winter squash, corn, peas, beans and lentils. Cut out high-sugar fruits such as apples, pears, bananas, stone fruits, oranges, dried fruit and fruit juices.

While most nuts and seeds are low in carbohydrates, higher-carb peanuts, soybeans, cashews and pistachios should be eaten sparingly. Finally, eliminate added sugars in drinks, condiments, desserts, baked goods and processed foods – these sugars creep up anywhere from sweetened yoghurts to ketchup to salad dressings. Terms like "corn syrup," "evaporated cane juice" and "fructose" on ingredient labels indicate added sugars, so read carefully before consuming.

CAN I EAT *ANY* CARBS?

You can consume 5 to 10 per cent of your daily calories from carbs while following a ketogenic diet. According to the Harvard School of Public Health, staying in ketosis requires keeping carbohydrates under 50 grams per day – the amount in a cup of pasta or rice. Depending on total caloric intake and activity level, you may need to reduce carbs further, to 20 or 30 grams. If you engage in high-intensity exercise that burns up glucose stores, you can likely consume a few more grams of carbohydrates while remaining in ketosis.

The *kinds* of carbs you eat also matters. Grains like wheat, rice and oats, along with simple sugars found in high-fructose fruits, corn syrup and table sugar, raise blood sugar quickly and significantly. This tells your body to use glucose rather than fat as fuel – taking you out of ketosis. Berries and non-starchy vegetables are better choices that won't cause blood sugar to spike.

WHAT ARE THE BENEFITS?

The keto diet has a well-documented ability to promote weight loss: A study published in *Nutrition Research* found participants in a 12-week keto diet lost an average of 18 kilograms (40 pounds) for men and 11 kilograms (24 pounds) for women. A *PubMed* analysis of 13 studies determined that dieters lost about two kilograms more on keto versus a low-fat diet. In addition, keto dieters lowered blood pressure and harmful LDL (low-density lipoprotein, or "bad") cholesterol.

According to research at the University of California San Francisco, by stopping glucose metabolism, the keto diet decreases inflammatory gene activity. The result? Reduced body and brain inflammation. This protects brain health, aids recovery from strokes, treats epilepsy and controls blood sugar spikes in Type 2 diabetes.

The ketogenic diet may even ward off cancer by starving tumours of sugars they need to grow. An analysis of 17 animal studies demonstrated that keto diets reduced the size of cancerous tumours.

IS IT SAFE?

Multiple studies demonstrate that following a keto diet for several months is a safe way to lose weight while obtaining ample energy to power the brain and body. In keto, this energy simply comes from fats rather than sugars. However, the effects of remaining in ketosis for more than six months haven't been adequately studied, so the diet is best used short-term.

Although keto is generally safe, the diet can be problematic for those with thyroid, kidney, gallbladder or pancreas conditions. Eating keto increases demands on these organs and can overstrain an already vulnerable system. In addition, keto is not suitable for pregnant and nursing women, as babies need carbohydrates to develop and grow.

> Check with your doctor before beginning and while following a keto diet to make sure you remain healthy.

ARE THERE ANY SIDE EFFECTS?

In the first week of a keto diet, many experience a "keto flu" consisting of headaches, stomach upset, fatigue and/or brain fog. While the exact cause of "keto flu" is unclear, research at the University of California San Francisco suggests electrolyte loss may be the culprit. Symptoms generally fade within a week or two as your body adjusts to ketosis.

In some cases, lack of electrolytes causes longer-lasting or more serious side effects, including muscle cramps and elevated heart rate. If these occur, stop the diet and seek advice from your doctor.

Because keto contains more fat and less fibre than an average diet, eating keto can cause gastrointestinal distress but symptoms often dissipate as your digestive system adapts.

Consult your doctor if any of the symptoms listed here are severe, or last longer than a week or two.

WHAT IS KETO BREATH?

While in ketosis, many dieters notice a distinctly acidic smell to their breath or metallic taste in their mouth – a phenomenon known as "keto breath." The taste and odour are a direct result of ketone production, as excess ketones are released through the breath. One of these ketones is acetone, the main ingredient in nail polish remover, and many describe keto breath as resembling the scent of nail polish remover.

Keto breath can also be caused by increased protein consumption. While digesting protein, your body produces ammonia, which is emitted through the breath. Like acetone, ammonia has a distinctively chemical taste and scent.

Keto breath is not dangerous, and it will likely fade once your body adapts to ketosis. In the meantime, you can manage unpleasant breath by eating less protein, brushing teeth regularly, using mouthwash and chewing sugar-free gum and mints.

ARE THERE DIFFERENT TYPES OF KETO DIETS?

The **standard keto** diet – which this book focuses on – contains 70 to 80 per cent calories from fat, 15 to 25 per cent from protein and 5 to 10 per cent from carbohydrates. However, other forms of keto vary these percentages.

Targeted keto, for those who exercise intensely and/ or for long periods, allows dieters to eat about 25 additional grams of carbs 30 to 45 minutes before physical activity. These carbs fuel athletic performance, but are burned off so ketosis resumes post-workout.

High-protein keto for bodybuilders boosts protein intake for muscle repair and growth. This version reduces fat to 65 per cent of calories while raising protein to 30 per cent, keeping carbs at only 5 per cent.

Keto cycling consists of a standard keto diet for 5 days, followed by a day or two with more carbs. This satisfies carb cravings and makes the diet easier to maintain over time.

IS IT SUITABLE FOR VEGANS AND VEGETARIANS?

The keto diet can be a healthy choice for vegetarians and vegans. In fact, a meat and/or dairy-free version of keto may be *more* beneficial, as avoiding animal products also bypasses the saturated fat these foods contain. According to the World Health Organization, you can protect heart health by reducing saturated fats from meat and dairy in favour of unsaturated fats from vegetable oils, nuts, seeds and avocados – all of which happen to be vegan.

Since meatless meals often rely on non-keto legumes, grains and high-carb vegetables, vegetarians must plan carefully to ensure their keto diet contains adequate protein and nutrients. Vegans eating keto can obtain protein from tofu, most nuts and seeds and keto-friendly protein powders. Vegetarians may add dairy and eggs as well.

Vegetarian/vegan keto dieters can also supplement with a multivitamin to ensure they're receiving all essential vitamins and minerals. See page 26 for more information on supplements.

HOW LONG SHOULD I STAY ON THE DIET FOR?

Because the long-term effects of keto have not been adequately studied, doctors and dieticians recommend following a strict keto diet for no longer than six months. Within this limit, your specific time spent on keto will depend on individual goals. Many adopt a keto diet to lose weight, and both the Centers for Disease Control and Prevention (CDC) in the USA and the National Health Service (NHS) in the UK recommend losing 0.5 to 1 kilogram per week for safe, sustainable weight loss. Therefore, someone aiming to lose 10 kilograms would follow a keto diet for three to five months. If you are eating keto for anti-inflammatory benefits, you might remain on the diet for longer.

Dieticians also caution against suddenly stopping keto, which could lead to gastrointestinal distress and/or weight gain. Add healthy carbs gradually, starting with just one serving a day, and continue to avoid sugar and processed foods.

HOW DOES IT DIFFER TO OTHER LOW-CARB DIETS?

Unlike other low-carb diets, such as Atkins or Paleo, the goal of a ketogenic diet is to stay in ketosis and burn only fat for energy. To achieve this, keto dieters must keep their carb intake below 50 grams a day, while other low-carb diets can include up to 150 grams of carbohydrates daily. In addition, because of keto's emphasis on fat as fuel, the diet includes a larger percentage of calories from fat. Other low-carb plans contain more protein.

Generally speaking, keto is more restrictive than other low-carb diets. However, this restriction can lead to weight loss and health breakthroughs by completely changing the way your body uses food to make energy. After losing weight on keto, you may choose to adopt a less-strict but still low-carb plan for the long term.

HOW DO I MEASURE MY LEVELS OF KETOSIS?

You don't have to measure ketone levels – if you are restricting carbs and losing weight, you'll know your diet is working. However, you may choose to test ketones after a few days on the diet and/or continue to monitor levels about once a week to ensure you're on the right track. At-home methods measure ketones in blood, breath or urine, with varying costs and efficacy.

- The most expensive method is a blood ketone metre, which reads a blood sample to determine ketones per litre of blood, providing the most accurate measurements.
- Less expensive is a pen-size keto breath metre. This less precise but quick, portable method measures the quantity of the ketone acetone in your breath.
- The least expensive method is using urine strips, but these are also the least accurate way to test for ketosis. Strips change colour to indicate a greater concentration of ketones in urine but provide no numerical measurements.

WHAT CAN (AND CAN'T) I DRINK?

While on keto, drink plenty of water to stay hydrated and stave off the "keto flu". If plain water doesn't appeal, add lemon or lime slices or fresh mint, or purchase unsweetened flavoured waters. Avoid drinks with added sugars or artificial sweeteners like aspartame, which may affect blood sugar levels. Steer clear of high-sugar fruit juices as well.

For your caffeine fix, coffee and tea are both keto-friendly. If desired, use a safe, keto-approved sweetener, such as stevia or erythritol. For a creamy taste, add single cream. Unsweetened almond or coconut milk are also great choices, both with coffee or tea and on their own. High-sugar, low-fat dairy milk should be avoided.

You can consume low-carb alcohols, such as rum, vodka, gin, tequila, whisky, wine and light beer. If making a cocktail, choose sugar-free mixers such as sparkling water. Avoid regular beer, which is high in carbs.

CAN I EXERCISE WHILE ON THE KETO DIET?

You can absolutely exercise while on keto – in fact, doing so maximizes health gains and weight loss. Several studies, from sources including the *Journal of the International Society of Sports Nutrition*, have determined that the keto diet leads to increased fat burning during exercise, along with greater endurance.

Since high-intensity exercise relies on glucose to fuel muscles, it may prove difficult for dieters just beginning keto. Lower-intensity cardiovascular activities, such as walking, jogging or swimming, along with strength and flexibility training, are better choices for the first weeks of a keto diet. Once your body has adjusted to ketosis, you can incorporate higher-intensity workouts. One University of British Columbia study suggests that eating keto improves the body's response to HIIT (high-intensity interval training), helping athletes become stronger, faster.

> Consult with a doctor to ensure your exercise plan is safe for your body.

DO I NEED TO TAKE SUPPLEMENTS?

The supplements you take while on keto will depend on your health needs, the variety of foods you eat and your activity level. Almost everyone can benefit from an electrolyte supplement containing sodium, potassium and magnesium when starting a keto diet. A proper electrolyte balance will prevent "keto flu" symptoms like headaches and muscle aches, and is especially important if you're exercising intensely.

You may take digestive enzymes to help your body process the increased fats of the keto diet, along with fibre supplements to keep digestion regular.

If you're eating a wide variety of foods, you can certainly obtain all essential nutrients on a keto diet. However, if you find yourself relying on the same few meals or if you are vegetarian or vegan, consider supplementing with a multivitamin.

> Your doctor or nutritionist can help determine the right supplements for your needs.

ARE SNACKS ALLOWED?

Snacks are certainly allowed on keto! This diet relies on a balance of high fat, moderate protein and low carbohydrates throughout all meals but makes no requirements for *when* you eat. Snacks can provide an energy boost before or after a workout, or you can graze throughout the day rather than eating large meals. Just be mindful of total calorie consumption if your goal is to lose weight and, of course, keep your snacks low-carb.

If you want something to munch on, veggies like celery, cucumbers and peppers, along with berries, offer nutrients without many calories. If you're looking for a more substantial energy boost, there's no shortage of packaged keto bars and snack foods available to buy – but for a preservative-free, homemade option, try any of the countless variations on "fat bombs" in the "Snacks" section of this book (p.105).

SHOULD I SEE MY DOCTOR BEFORE STARTING THE DIET?

It's a good idea to see a doctor before starting any diet. This is especially true for keto, which significantly alters typical eating patterns and changes the way your body produces energy. A doctor can help you identify the foods and exercise routine that will keep you healthiest while in ketosis, and they can also manage any side effects.

Seeing a doctor is particularly important if you're taking medication for diabetes or high blood pressure. Since a keto diet can lower blood pressure and blood sugar, meds may need to be adjusted so these levels don't fall *too* low. In addition, a doctor can make sure you're not dealing with a health condition that makes a keto diet unsuitable.

Read more about the health conditions for which keto is *not* advisable on the next page.

WHEN IS THE KETO DIET NOT SAFE?

The keto diet is not safe for anyone with a kidney, gallbladder, pancreas or thyroid disease, as keto requires these organs to work harder. Eating keto increases the amount of uric acid to be processed by the kidneys, which may lead to kidney stones, while the gallbladder and pancreas must digest increased fat. Ketosis can also alter thyroid hormone levels, which could prove dangerous for those with thyroid conditions.

Keto is unsafe for pregnant and nursing women, as developing babies require both glucose and ample nutrients the mother might not obtain on a strict keto diet.

Finally, those with heart conditions should be careful not to eat too much saturated fat while on keto. According to the World Health Organization, excess saturated fat consumption may raise blood pressure and increase the risk of heart disease.

HOW DO I GET STARTED?

Just by picking up this book, you've taken the first steps toward adopting a ketogenic diet. You've learned what the keto diet entails, what foods to emphasize and avoid, how to measure levels of ketosis and what side effects and potential dangers to look out for. In the remainder of this guide, you'll find keto recipes for every meal of the day and a two-week meal planner to guide you on your journey.

> You should consult your doctor before beginning keto, and consider visiting a nutritionist for extra support.

Once you've decided to try keto, ensure you have ample keto-friendly foods at home and get rid of high-carb temptations if possible. Making a meal plan for your first weeks of keto will set you up for success.

Finally, take time to enjoy your delicious keto meals and celebrate every health gain along the way!

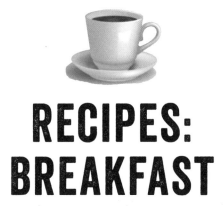

RECIPES:
BREAKFAST

SOME CLASSIC BREAKFAST FOODS, LIKE
HIGH-FAT, LOW-CARB EGGS AND BACON,
ARE A NATURAL FIT FOR A KETO DIET. ON
THE OTHER HAND, YOU MIGHT BE WORRIED
ABOUT GIVING UP TOAST, PANCAKES,
CEREALS AND FRUIT SMOOTHIES – BUT
WITH THE RECIPES IN THIS CHAPTER, YOU
CAN STILL ENJOY SWEET MORNING TREATS.

READ ON TO FIND OPTIONS FOR QUICK
MORNING MEALS AND LEISURELY WEEKEND
BRUNCHES, ALL LOW IN CARBS AND HIGH
IN HEALTHY FATS AND NUTRIENTS.

EGGS WITH KALE, MUSHROOMS AND TOMATO

SERVES SIX (VEGETARIAN)

This hearty, vegetarian egg dish provides healthy fats and protein to fuel you for the day ahead. It's savoury and satisfying enough to work for a quick supper as well. You can substitute spinach or Swiss chard for kale, leave out mushrooms or tomato if you don't have them on hand, or serve with avocado for additional healthy fats and nutrients.

INGREDIENTS

2 tbsp butter or olive oil, or 1 tbsp of each

180 g (6½ oz) assorted mushrooms,
sliced – button, cremini, portobello
or shiitake will all work

140 g (5 oz) fresh kale, torn into
bite-sized pieces

1 medium fresh tomato, chopped

2 tbsp chopped fresh herbs or 1 tsp dried –
rosemary, thyme and sage are great options

6 eggs

salt and pepper

METHOD

Heat the butter and/or olive oil in a large frying pan over a medium-high heat. (If combining butter and oil, heat the butter first to give it time to melt.) Add the mushrooms and sauté until they begin to turn brown (about 3–5 minutes).

Add the kale, herbs, and salt and pepper to taste. Cook until the kale wilts (about 3 minutes) then add the tomato and cook for 1 minute more.

Make six wells in the vegetable mixture, and add a small amount of butter or oil to each well. Crack the eggs into open spaces, sprinkle with additional salt and pepper, cover with a lid and cook until the egg yolks are runny or firm according to your taste (about 2–4 minutes).

Remove from heat and serve warm. Leftovers can be covered with plastic wrap, refrigerated for up to 2–3 days and reheated in the microwave or oven.

KETO PUMPKIN PANCAKES WITH COCONUT CREAM

SERVES SIX TO EIGHT (VEGETARIAN)

Yes, you can enjoy pancakes on a keto diet – just use low-carb almond flour in your batter. The addition of pumpkin turns these pancakes into an extra-special, vegetarian autumn treat. Although winter squash is too high in carbs to be eaten regularly on keto, this recipe contains just enough pumpkin to add that seasonal flavour you might be craving.

INGREDIENTS

4 eggs

120 g (4 oz) full-fat cream cheese

170 g (6 oz) almond flour

112 g (4 oz) unsweetened canned pumpkin or mashed baked pumpkin

2 tbsp keto-friendly granulated sweetener

1 tsp maple extract

1 tbsp cinnamon

½ tsp ginger

¼ tsp cloves

¼ tsp nutmeg

1 tsp baking powder

dash of salt

1 tbsp butter

Optional ingredients for coconut cream topping:

1 can (425 g/15 oz) coconut cream, stored in refrigerator overnight

keto-friendly sweetener, cinnamon and maple extract to taste

METHOD

If serving with coconut cream, prepare this first by placing the chilled canned coconut cream in a large bowl. Beat with an electric mixer until light and fluffy, then add the sweetener and optional cinnamon and/or maple extract to taste.

For the pancake batter, beat the eggs in a large mixing bowl with a metal whisk, then add cream cheese, almond flour, pumpkin, sweetener, maple extract, spices, baking powder and salt and whisk until combined. Alternatively, place all the ingredients in blender or food processor and blend into a smooth batter.

Melt the butter in a large frying pan over a medium heat. Add 50 grams (2 ounces) batter to the pan. Cook until bubbles form in centre of pancake, then flip and cook until firm and light brown. Repeat until all the batter is used.

Serve the pancakes warm, with coconut cream if desired. Leftover pancakes can be covered and refrigerated for five days or frozen in a Ziploc bag for up to two months. Reheat in the microwave or on the stovetop.

KETO BERRY PORRIDGE

SERVES ONE (VEGAN)

Porridge (or oatmeal) is a classic stick-to-your-ribs breakfast... which contains too many carbs for a keto diet. However, this keto version may be even more satisfying with the addition of healthy fats from flax, coconut, chia and hemp. This recipe is also a great vegan source of protein, vitamins and minerals.

Experiment with different combinations of spices (try cinnamon, ginger or nutmeg) and berries to keep your taste buds guessing.

INGREDIENTS

120 ml (4 fl oz) unsweetened coconut milk

2 tbsp hemp seeds

2 tbsp ground flaxseeds

1 tbsp chia seeds

1 tbsp unsweetened shredded coconut

1 tsp stevia or other granulated keto-friendly sweetener

½ tsp cardamom

¼ tsp fresh lemon zest

pinch of salt

40 g (1½ oz) blueberries, blackberries, raspberries, sliced strawberries or combination

METHOD

You can cook this in a pan on the stove or in the microwave.

If you are preparing on a stove:

Add all the ingredients except for the berries to a small saucepan. Cook over a low heat for 3–5 minutes, stirring constantly, until thick.

If you are using a microwave:

Combine all the ingredients except for the berries in a microwave-safe bowl. Microwave on high for 2 minutes, then stir.

For both methods, top the porridge with berries and serve warm.

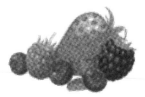

BACON, EGG AND BROCCOLI "MUFFINS"

SERVES SIX

Broccoli for breakfast? When it's part of a delicious eggy "muffin," you bet! The portable shape makes these perfect for a grab-and-go breakfast, especially if you make and freeze the "muffins" ahead of time.

INGREDIENTS

4 slices bacon

7 eggs

180 g (6½ oz) broccoli, chopped
into bite-size pieces

½ tsp paprika

½ tsp salt

¼ tsp pepper

1 tbsp almond or coconut flour

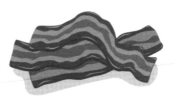

METHOD

Cook the bacon until it is nice and crispy, either by pan-frying for 5-6 minutes or baking in the oven at 200°C (400°F) for 15-20 minutes. When the bacon has cooled, crumble it into small pieces.

For the egg muffins, preheat the oven to 200°C (400°F). Grease a six-muffin pan with butter or add paper liners.

In a medium mixing bowl, beat one egg. Add the broccoli, paprika, salt, pepper and flour and stir until the broccoli is coated.

Place 2 tablespoons of the broccoli mixture in the bottom of each muffin cup and press down. Bake for 10 minutes, then remove from the oven.

Sprinkle 1 teaspoon of bacon on each muffin, then crack one egg over each. Bake for 20 minutes, cool for 5 minutes then remove from the pan. Serve warm or store in the fridge in an airtight container for up to five days, or freeze for up to two months. Reheat in the microwave to serve.

ALL-PURPOSE
KETO SMOOTHIE

SERVES ONE (VEGAN)

On a busy morning, there's nothing better than a smoothie that you can pour into a cup and take with you. This all-purpose, vegan recipe allows for endless smoothie variations, from Raspberry Coconut to Blueberry Chia to Strawberry Spinach, and will really fuel you up for the day. Your creativity is the only limit here!

INGREDIENTS

160 g (5½ oz) frozen strawberries, blueberries, blackberries, raspberries or any combination

70 g (2½ oz) fresh kale, spinach, Swiss chard or any combination

240 ml (8¼ fl oz) unsweetened coconut or almond milk

Optional additions:

1 small avocado, peeled and mashed

2 tbsp unsweetened shredded coconut

2 tbsp unsweetened dark chocolate chips

2 tbsp chia seeds

2 tbsp hemp seeds

1 tsp vanilla extract

1 tsp lemon zest

METHOD

Place your chosen combination of berries, greens, milk and any additions into a blender. Blend until combined and smooth.

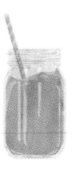

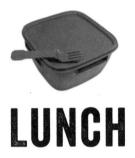

LUNCH

FROM PIZZA TO SANDWICH WRAPS, MAC
AND CHEESE TO TACOS — WITH THE
LOW-CARB VERSIONS IN THIS CHAPTER,
YOU DON'T HAVE TO GIVE UP DELICIOUS
LUNCHTIME DISHES. YOU'LL FIND QUICK
RECIPES TO PREPARE AHEAD AND BRING TO
WORK, PORTABLE OPTIONS FOR A PICNIC
AND SPECIAL TREATS FIT FOR A PARTY.

MINI CABBAGE CRUST PIZZAS

SERVES SIX

Sliced cabbage rounds make the perfect low-carb substitute for traditional pizza dough, and baking the cabbage "crust" transforms its bitter flavour to a sweeter one. This recipe is vegetarian, unless you choose to add meat pizza toppings like crumbled bacon, chopped ham or pepperoni.

INGREDIENTS

½ medium red cabbage

salt and pepper

240 g (8½ oz) canned crushed/chopped tomatoes

1 tbsp red wine vinegar

1 tsp dried oregano

1 large ball of fresh mozzarella cheese, thinly sliced

keto-friendly pizza toppings of choice (sliced olives, sliced green peppers, crumbled bacon, pepperoni, chopped ham, etc.)

1 tbsp olive oil

2 tbsp fresh chopped basil, oregano or a combination

METHOD

Preheat oven to 190°C (375°F).

Remove the outer leaves from the cabbage, then slice it into six rounds of about 1 centimetre thickness. Place the rounds on a baking sheet and sprinkle lightly with salt and pepper.

Combine the tomatoes, vinegar and dried oregano and spread evenly over the cabbage. Cover with thinly sliced cheese and other toppings of your choice. Drizzle with olive oil.

Bake for 20-25 minutes, or until the cheese is melted and light brown. Sprinkle with fresh herbs and serve warm.

Store leftovers in the fridge, covered, for up to three days, and enjoy warm or cold.

BACON, LETTUCE AND TOMATO WRAPS

SERVES TWO

This low-carb version of the classic BLT is not only lower in calories, it's also more portable and easier to eat, thanks to the lettuce wrap shape. You can also add sliced cheese or avocado, and once you get the hang of making lettuce wraps, experiment with a variety of sandwich fillings.

INGREDIENTS

4 strips cooked bacon or turkey
bacon, cut in half

2 small heads iceberg lettuce, cored,
outer leaves discarded

2 tbsp sugar-free mayonnaise

1 tsp red wine vinegar

4 slices tomato

salt and pepper

METHOD

Cook the bacon until just starting to crisp by pan-frying for 4–6 minutes or baking in the oven at 200°C (400°F) for 12–15 minutes.

Lay one sheet of parchment or waxed paper, about 30 by 30 centimetres (12 by 12 inches), flat on a work surface. Arrange five to eight large lettuce leaves in the centre of the paper, so they overlap. If the lettuce is breaking into smaller pieces, add some extra layers.

Combine the mayonnaise and vinegar and spread half the mixture on the lettuce. Top with two slices of bacon and tomato and season with salt and pepper to taste.

Roll the lettuce as tightly as possible, and when completely wrapped, roll the paper around the lettuce to keep it together until it is ready to eat. Repeat to make second sandwich.

Slice in half with serrated knife and enjoy.

AVOCADO AND EGG SALAD

SERVES TWO AS A MAIN DISH,
FOUR AS A SIDE (VEGETARIAN)

Thanks to the addition of protein-rich eggs, this refreshing, summery salad is satisfying enough to serve as a vegetarian lunch on its own. You can omit the eggs or substitute crumbled tofu for a vegan option.

This salad tastes best after chilling for several hours, so it's a great make-ahead option – especially on hot days when you don't want to turn on the oven.

INGREDIENTS

4 hard-boiled eggs, peeled and chopped, or 130 g (4½ oz) crumbled tofu if you are making this as a vegan meal

2 ripe but firm avocados, cut into 1 cm (0.4 in.) cubes

1 large or 2 small cucumbers, chopped into 1 cm (0.4 in.) cubes

1 large tomato, chopped into 1 cm (0.4 in.) cubes

1 green pepper, diced

2 tbsp chopped red onion

2 tbsp chopped fresh parsley, chives, and/or coriander

2 tbsp olive oil

juice of one lime

salt and cayenne pepper to taste

METHOD

In a large serving bowl, combine the eggs (or tofu), avocado, cucumber, tomato, green pepper, red onion and herbs.

Mix the olive oil and lime juice in a small bowl or cup, then drizzle over the vegetables and stir to combine. Top with salt and pepper to taste, and an additional garnish of fresh herbs.

Serve immediately, or cover and refrigerate for several hours to let the flavours meld before enjoying. Any leftovers can be refrigerated up to two days.

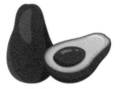

KETO CAULIFLOWER
MAC AND CHEESE

SERVES FOUR TO SIX (VEGETARIAN)

Cauliflower provides a satisfying substitute for pasta in this keto "mac" and cheese dish. You can experiment with different cheeses, using shredded Parmesan or mozzarella in place of some or all of the cheddar. Use half broccoli, half cauliflower for a stronger vegetable flavour.

While this dish is vegetarian (as long as you use vegetarian cheese), you can sprinkle crumbled bacon bits on top before grilling for a non-veggie version.

INGREDIENTS

1 tsp salt

600 g (1 lb 3 oz) chopped
cauliflower, or use half cauliflower
and half broccoli

1 tbsp butter

2 tbsp finely chopped onion

2 tbsp finely chopped chives, optional

2 tbsp almond flour

350 ml (12 fl oz) unsweetened almond
or cashew milk

2 tbsp single cream

1 tsp nutritional yeast

80 g (3 oz) finely shredded
cheddar cheese

METHOD

Preheat oven to 205°C (400°F).

Pour water in a large pot to a depth of 3 centimetres (1.2 inches) and add half a teaspoon of salt. Bring to a boil, add the cauliflower and cook over a medium heat until tender but still firm (about 6 minutes). Remove from heat and drain.

Melt the butter in a saucepan over a medium heat, add the onion and sauté for 2 minutes, then add the chives and cook for an additional 30 seconds. Lower the heat, stir in the almond flour and cook for 3 minutes. Raise heat to medium, add the milk and cream and bring to a boil, whisking constantly. Add half a teaspoon of salt and the nutritional yeast. Remove from the heat and gradually stir in the cheese until melted.

Fold the cauliflower into the cheese sauce, place in 20 by 20 centimetres (8 by 8 inches) baking dish, and bake for 15-20 minutes until golden. Place under a grill for 2 minutes and serve.

Refrigerate any leftovers in an airtight container for up to three days and reheat in the microwave.

MEXICAN STUFFED AVOCADOS

SERVES FOUR

This easy recipe makes a delicious taco-style meal without the carbs of a tortilla. It's equally suitable for a casual lunch or a fiesta.

You can substitute shredded turkey or ground/minced beef for the chicken. If you have some cooked, seasoned meat left over, you can use it to make taco salad by combining with veggies and cheese.

INGREDIENTS

juice of 1 lime
or lemon

4 ripe but firm
avocados, halved
and pitted

1 tbsp olive oil

1 small onion,
chopped

450 g (1 lb) skinless
chicken breast

2 tbsp tomato paste

1 tbsp chilli powder

½ tsp salt

¼ tsp garlic powder

¼ tsp onion powder

35 g (1¼ oz) shredded
iceberg or romaine
lettuce

1 small tomato,
chopped

4 tbsp sliced black
olives (about 8 olives)

40 g (1½ oz) grated/
shredded Gouda
(or other mild
hard cheese)

2 tbsp chopped fresh
coriander

4 tbsp sour cream

METHOD

Sprinkle lime or lemon juice over the avocado halves to prevent browning and set them on a serving platter.

Heat the oil in a large frying pan over a medium heat. Sauté the onion for 5 minutes or until soft and translucent, then set aside. Place chicken breast in pan, cook for 5 minutes, turn over, cover with water and cook for another 7-10 minutes. Remove from heat and shred the chicken by either using two forks to separate and shred meat, or placing in a food mixer and using the flat beater attachment for about 15 seconds. Combine the chicken and onion, then stir in the tomato paste and seasonings.

Fill the avocado halves with chicken, then top with lettuce, tomato and olives, sprinkle with cheese and coriander, and finish with a spoonful of sour cream.

This dish is best served immediately so the avocado doesn't brown, but leftover meat can be refrigerated in an airtight container for three days.

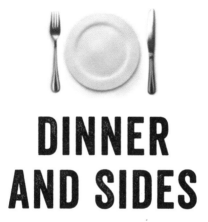

DINNER
AND SIDES

IN THIS CHAPTER, YOU'LL FIND DINNER
OPTIONS RANGING FROM SOUPS TO SALADS,
DECADENT BUTTER CHICKEN TO BEEF
STIR-FRY, AND LOW-CARB TAKES ON RICE
AND MASHED POTATOES. READ ON FOR
FILLING MAIN DISHES FEATURING BEEF,
CHICKEN, PORK, SALMON AND A VEGAN
OPTION, ALONG WITH A VARIETY OF SIDES.

BROCCOLI-CAULIFLOWER KETO SOUP

SERVES SIX

This twist on the classic broccoli
cheddar soup is filling enough
to serve as a light supper
on its own, perhaps with a
side of the flatbread included
later in this chapter (page 94).
It's also delicious with
salad or veggie sides. Omit
the bacon to transform this
into a vegetarian meal.

INGREDIENTS

4 strips bacon

½ onion, diced

2 carrots, diced

4 stalks celery, diced

2 tbsp chives, diced

180 g (6½ oz)
broccoli, chopped
into bite-sized pieces

180 g (6½ oz)
cauliflower, chopped
into bite-sized pieces

185 g (6½ oz)
chopped courgette

480 ml (16 fl oz)
single or whipping
cream

480 ml (16 fl oz)
vegetable stock

240 g (8½ oz) finely
grated cheddar cheese

4 tbsp cream cheese

1 tsp paprika

salt and pepper

METHOD

Place the bacon in bottom of large soup pot over a medium heat and cook until crisp (5–10 minutes), turning once. Remove the bacon from the pot, let the bacon cool and then crumble it into small pieces.

While the bacon is cooling, add the onions, carrots and celery to the pot. Sauté until soft (about 8 minutes), then add the chives and cook for another minute.

Add the broccoli, cauliflower, courgette, cream and stock to the pot, and increase the heat until the liquid reaches a simmer. Cook uncovered for 5–10 minutes until veggies are tender, stirring frequently. Gradually add the grated cheese and the cream cheese and stir until all the cheese is melted.

Simmer the soup until thick, about 10 more minutes, stirring frequently. Season with paprika and salt and pepper to taste. Spoon into bowls and top with bacon crumbles and additional chives.

Store leftover soup in an airtight container and refrigerate for up to five days or freeze for up to two months.

KETO BEEF AND BROCCOLI STIR-FRY

SERVES FOUR TO SIX

This hearty meal will remind you of your favourite Chinese takeaway, but without all those pesky sugars and carbs often added to restaurant fare. If you find yourself missing rice on the side, serve with cauliflower rice.

INGREDIENTS

2 tbsp coconut oil
or olive oil

2 tsp fresh ginger,
grated

1 clove fresh garlic,
crushed

140 ml (5 fl oz)
soy sauce or liquid
aminos

2 tbsp cider vinegar

675 g (1 lb 8 oz) skirt
steak, sliced against
the grain into thin,
bite-sized strips

2 tbsp sesame oil

720 g (1 lb 9 oz)
broccoli florets,
chopped into bite-
sized pieces

1 green pepper,
chopped into bite-
sized pieces

2 tbsp sesame seeds

salt and pepper

METHOD

In a large bowl, whisk together the coconut or olive oil (if the coconut oil has solidified, melt it for a few seconds in a microwave), ginger, garlic, soy sauce or aminos, and vinegar. Add the meat, stir to coat thoroughly, cover and marinate for several hours in the refrigerator.

Heat 1 tablespoon of sesame oil in a large frying pan over a high heat. Add the steak in a single layer and top with half the sauce, sear for 3 minutes, turn, and cook for 2-3 more minutes.

Add the remaining sesame oil, broccoli, pepper and remaining sauce. Stir-fry for about 10 minutes, until the veggies are tender. Add sesame seeds and salt and pepper to taste, cook for another minute, then remove from heat and serve.

Refrigerate leftovers in an airtight container for three to four days or freeze for two to three months. Thaw in the fridge overnight before reheating and serving.

KETO BUTTER CHICKEN

SERVES FOUR

This Indian-inspired dish is particularly delicious and healthy when made with ghee, or Indian clarified butter. Ghee is full of fat-soluble vitamins and fatty acids that have anti-inflammatory effects on the body.

Serve this dish with broccoli or cauliflower rice (page 88) or keto flatbread (page 94).

INGREDIENTS

450 g (1 lb) chicken breast,
cut into bite-size cubes

1 tbsp garam masala

1 tsp turmeric powder

1 tsp grated ginger

1 tsp minced garlic

½ tsp salt

125 g (4½ oz) unsweetened whole
milk Greek yoghurt

2 tbsp butter or ghee

1 small yellow onion, chopped

180 ml (6 fl oz) whipping cream

1.5 tbsp tomato paste

handful of fresh parsley

METHOD

In a large bowl, coat the chicken cubes with garam masala, turmeric, ginger, garlic and salt. Stir in the yoghurt, cover and refrigerate for at least half an hour.

Heat the butter or ghee in a large frying pan over a medium-high heat, add the onion and cook for 3 minutes or until translucent. Meanwhile, remove the chicken from the marinade and discard the yoghurt mixture. Add the chicken to the pan and cook for 6 minutes, turning once.

Reduce heat to medium-low, stir in the whipping cream and tomato paste, cover and cook for 5–7 minutes until the chicken is cooked through and has reached the desired tenderness. Remove from the heat, garnish with parsley and serve.

Refrigerate leftovers in an airtight container for three to four days, or freeze for up to six months and let thaw in the fridge overnight before reheating.

PORK CHOPS WITH MUSHROOMS

SERVES FOUR

Pork chops make for a hearty, fat- and protein-rich dinner. Choose chops with a fatty cut for the juiciest flavour. You can substitute the mushrooms or add other vegetables – asparagus, green beans (one of the only keto-friendly beans!) or green peppers would all work well.

INGREDIENTS

8 tbsp butter or olive oil

2 garlic cloves, minced

1 tsp dried rosemary

1 tsp dried thyme

salt and pepper

4 medium pork chops

180 g (6½ oz) sliced button or cremini mushrooms

2 tbsp chives, chopped

METHOD

Melt the butter or heat the olive oil in a large frying pan over a medium heat. Add the garlic and cook for 2–3 minutes until beginning to brown, then add the rosemary, thyme and a sprinkle of salt and pepper.

Cut a few slices in the surface of the pork chops to release steam, add to the pan and cook for 5–10 minutes per side (depending on the thickness of the chops), until they are done all the way through.

Remove the pork chops from the pan, add the mushrooms and an additional shake of salt and pepper, and sauté for 5–6 minutes until browned, adding chives in the final minute.

Pour the mushrooms and remaining butter or oil mixture over pork chops and serve.

Store leftovers in the fridge in an airtight container for up to three days.

CRISPY AND CREAMY PARMESAN SALMON

SERVES FOUR

Salmon provides plenty of heart-healthy fats and is one of the richest dietary sources of omega 3 fatty acids – which makes it a perfect choice for keto! This salmon recipe is quick and easy to prepare and delicious with any vegetable side dish, such as the Roasted Green Beans later in this chapter (page 91).

INGREDIENTS

4 x 225 g (8 oz) salmon fillets

1 lemon, juiced

½ tsp salt

4 tbsp sour cream

1 tsp lemon zest

2 tbsp chopped fresh sage

2 cloves garlic, minced

8 tbsp grated Parmesan cheese

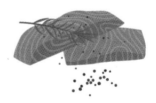

METHOD

Preheat oven to 220°C (425°F). Line a large baking sheet with parchment paper.

Arrange the four salmon fillets on a baking sheet and pour lemon juice over the top, reserving 1 tablespoon for later. Sprinkle with salt.

In a small bowl, stir together the sour cream, lemon zest, sage, garlic and half the cheese. Spread the mixture evenly over the salmon.

Sprinkle additional cheese on top of the sour cream mixture.

Bake in the oven for 15-20 minutes until cooked all the way through, then drizzle with reserved lemon juice and serve.

Wrap any leftover salmon tightly in foil, place in a sealed container and refrigerate for up to four days. Reheat in the oven to serve.

COURGETTE "SPAGHETTI" WITH HEMP AND HERB PESTO

SERVES FOUR TO SIX (VEGAN)

This completely vegan main dish uses hemp seeds (often sold as "hemp hearts") as the basis for a pesto that is rich in protein, omega 3, vitamins and minerals and is also full of flavour. Feel free to add other keto-friendly vegetables or garnishes, such as olives or chopped almonds, to your taste.

INGREDIENTS

80 g (3 oz) hemp
seeds, hulled

1 tbsp nutritional
yeast

¼ tsp salt

1 clove garlic, crushed

70 g (2½ oz) fresh
spinach

35 g (1¼ oz) fresh
parsley

35 g (1¼ oz) fresh
basil

2 tbsp olive oil

2 tbsp lemon juice

720 g (1 lb 9 oz)
spiralized courgette
– either buy prepared
or use a spiralizer

150 g (5 oz) cherry
tomatoes, halved

1 avocado, cut into
bite-sized cubes,
optional

METHOD

Place the hemp seeds, nutritional yeast, salt, garlic, spinach, parsley, basil, olive oil and lemon juice in a blender or food processor and blend until smooth.

In a large bowl, pour the pesto over the courgette noodles and stir until thoroughly coated. Add the tomatoes and avocado (if using) and fold in until evenly mixed. Serve immediately.

Refrigerate leftovers in an airtight container for three to four days. Extra pesto will stay fresh in the fridge for up to a week, or freeze in an airtight container for up to six months.

CAULIFLOWER MASH

SERVES FOUR (VEGETARIAN)

Perhaps one of the most-missed foods on a keto diet is potatoes – but you don't have to give up a creamy, buttery, garlicky mash while on keto! Cauliflower provides a lower-carb, lower-calorie and nutrient-rich substitute for potatoes.

Buttermilk will add a tangier flavour to this recipe, while single cream will be creamier. You can omit the liquid for a thicker mash and substitute vegan butter and cream cheese for a vegan version.

INGREDIENTS

1 medium head cauliflower,
cut into small pieces

2 cloves garlic, peeled

1 tbsp cream cheese

1 tbsp butter

60 ml (2 fl oz) buttermilk or single cream

$\frac{1}{2}$ tsp salt

$\frac{1}{4}$ tsp black pepper

METHOD

Boil or steam the cauliflower and garlic until soft for 7-9 minutes.

Remove from the heat, drain and separate out and mash the garlic cloves.

Combine all the ingredients in a large bowl and puree with an immersion blender, or place in a regular blender or food processor and puree until smooth.

Serve while still warm, perhaps with more butter on top. Refrigerate leftovers in an airtight container for up to three days.

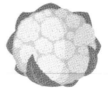

BROCCOLI "RICE"

SERVES FOUR (VEGAN)

You've probably heard of cauliflower "rice" – but you can also make a delicious rice substitute with broccoli! Of course, if you want to use cauliflower or even chopped courgette or summer squash in this recipe, you can do so as well.

INGREDIENTS

1 large head of broccoli, cut into bite-size pieces

1 tbsp olive or avocado oil

2 tbsp chopped onion

2 cloves garlic, diced

½ tsp salt

¼ tsp pepper

1 tbsp lime juice

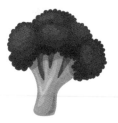

METHOD

Use a food processor to pulse the broccoli into tiny, rice grain-sized pieces. If you don't have a food processor, you can chop the broccoli by hand or buy it pre-riced.

Heat the oil in a medium pan over a medium heat. Add the onion and garlic and cook for 2 minutes, then add the broccoli, salt, pepper and lime juice. Cook for 1–2 minutes, until tender but still crunchy and firm. Serve warm. Store leftovers in the fridge in an airtight container for up to three days.

ROASTED GREEN BEANS WITH CHERRY TOMATOES AND ALMONDS

SERVES SIX (VEGAN)

Green beans are one of the only low-carb legumes, which makes them perfect for a keto side dish! This recipe is vegan, but you can also top with shredded Parmesan cheese and bake for a few additional minutes until the cheese melts.

INGREDIENTS

250 g (9 oz) fresh green beans, stems removed

2 tbsp avocado oil or olive oil

1 tsp garlic powder

1 tsp salt

¼ tsp black pepper

150 g (5 oz) cherry tomatoes, halved

23 g (¾ oz) sliced almonds

2 tbsp lemon zest

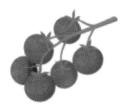

METHOD

Preheat oven to 200°C (400°F). Line a baking sheet with parchment paper.

Arrange the green beans on the parchment paper, drizzle with oil, sprinkle with garlic powder, salt and pepper, and toss with a wooden spoon so that all the beans are evenly coated with the oil and seasoning.

Bake for 15 minutes.

Remove from the oven, toss the beans again, add the cherry tomatoes and then sprinkle the almonds and lemon zest over the top. Bake for an additional 10 minutes and serve.

Cover leftovers and refrigerate for up to three days.

CHEESY KETO FLATBREAD

SERVES FOUR

While following a keto diet, you might miss having bread with your dinner – but with a recipe this easy to whip up, you can make keto flatbread to accompany any meal! Most keto cooks agree that this is the best way to make low-carb flatbreads. It's especially good paired with soup or salad, like the Broccoli-Cauliflower Keto Soup in this chapter (page 67).

INGREDIENTS

80 g (3 oz) finely shredded mozzarella cheese

1 tbsp cream cheese, softened

1 egg

28 g (1 oz) almond flour

¼ tsp Italian seasoning or garlic powder,
optional

¼ tsp salt

METHOD

Preheat oven to 180°C (350°F). Line a baking sheet with parchment paper.

Combine the mozzarella and cream cheeses in a small, microwave-safe bowl and heat in 15-second bursts, stirring between each one, until melted and smooth. Alternatively, place the cheeses in a saucepan and heat until melted, stirring frequently.

While the cheeses cool (after about 5 minutes), beat the egg in another bowl and stir in the almond flour and seasonings.

Add half the melted cheese to the almond flour and egg mixture, fold in gently, then add the remaining cheese and combine thoroughly.

Divide the dough into four balls, space evenly on the baking sheet and press into flatbreads.

Bake for 15–17 minutes until golden brown.

DESSERTS
AND SNACKS

MAKING YOUR OWN KETO SNACKS,
LIKE NUT-AND-SEED-PACKED
"FAT BOMBS", ENSURES YOU'RE
BYPASSING THE ARTIFICIAL INGREDIENTS
IN PACKAGED KETO SNACK FOODS.

AND DON'T FORGET DESSERT! WITH
THE HELP OF HIGH-FAT INGREDIENTS
LIKE CREAM CHEESE, WHIPPING
CREAM AND COCONUT, THE LOW-
CARB, LOW-SUGAR DESSERTS IN THIS
CHAPTER TASTE EVERY BIT AS SINFUL
AS TRADITIONAL SWEET TREATS!

SAVOURY AVOCADO DIP

SERVES FOUR TO SIX

(VEGETARIAN)

This delicious vegetarian dip gets a boost in healthy fat, vitamins B6, C and E, and magnesium from avocado, plus protein and calcium from yoghurt. Serve with low-carb veggies like celery, broccoli and cauliflower, or use as a spread on low-carb tortillas or pitas.

INGREDIENTS

2 ripe avocados

125 g (4½ oz) unsweetened whole
milk Greek yoghurt

2 tbsp cream cheese, at room temperature,
or sour cream

1 tsp fresh lemon juice

¼ tsp Dijon mustard

¼ tsp cayenne pepper

salt and black pepper to taste

2 tbsp chopped fresh dill

METHOD

Peel and pit the avocados. Mash lightly, then place in a food processor or blender along with all the ingredients except the dill. Puree until smooth and fully combined. Add 1½ tablespoons of dill and pulse until just incorporated.

Transfer to a serving bowl and garnish with the remaining dill. Serve with veggies or as a spread on low-carb pitas or tortillas.

Leftover dip can be kept in the fridge up to two days. To prevent the surface from browning, press plastic wrap onto the top of the dip and seal completely.

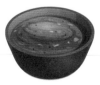

SALAD SKEWERS

SERVES EIGHT

Salad on a stick makes a perfect keto snack or appetizer! It's a fun (and attractive!) way to eat your veggies. Feel free to add any keto-friendly vegetables that will fit on a skewer.

INGREDIENTS

mini wooden skewers

16 cherry or grape tomatoes (use red, yellow and orange tomatoes for a rainbow skewer)

16 button mushrooms

8 large pitted black or green olives

16 mini mozzarella cheese balls

35 g (1¼ oz) spinach leaves

balsamic or red wine vinegar (to drizzle)

olive or avocado oil (to drizzle)

salt and pepper

METHOD

Thread the vegetables, cheese and spinach onto the skewers, alternating one or two spinach leaves between every other item. Use two tomatoes, two mushrooms, two cheese balls and one olive per skewer. If the spinach leaves are particularly large, fold in half or thirds.

Drizzle the skewers with vinegar and oil and sprinkle with salt and pepper. Serve immediately or refrigerate until ready to eat.

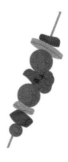

CUSTOMIZABLE
KETO "FAT BOMBS"

MAKES 12 FAT BOMBS (VEGETARIAN)

Keto fat bombs incorporate high-fat, high-nutrient nuts, seeds and nut butters into a bite-sized package. These concentrated sources of fat will give you energy, keep you in ketosis and satisfy your between-meal cravings.

INGREDIENTS

225 g (8 oz) assorted low-carb nuts – any combination of almonds, pecans, macadamia nuts, hazelnuts and Brazil nuts

125 g (4½ oz) unsweetened almond, pecan, sunflower seed or pumpkin seed butter

65 g (2¼ oz) keto powdered sugar

2 tbsp chia seeds, hemp seeds or flax seeds

2 tbsp unsweetened almond, coconut or cashew milk

Optional additions:

1–2 tbsp coconut oil

1–2 tbsp cream cheese

1–2 tbsp unsweetened cocoa powder

1 tsp cinnamon

1 tsp cardamom

METHOD

Place the nuts in a blender or food processor and pulse to a fine crumble. Add the nut or seed butter, keto sugar and seeds and blend until thoroughly combined, scraping down the sides of the blender or processor as necessary. Add the milk and optional additions and blend completely. If the mixture is too liquid, add more nut butter; if the mixture is too dry, add more milk.

Place in a bowl, cover and refrigerate for 30 minutes.

Once chilled, form the mixture into 12 equally sized balls. Cover and keep in the refrigerator for up to two weeks or freeze for up to six months.

KETO RASPBERRY-LEMON CHEESECAKE

SERVES 12

(VEGETARIAN)

With its base of creamy cheese and eggs rather than flour, cheesecake is a natural fit for a keto dessert. This version uses almond flour for a low-carb crust and adds a fruity and citrusy flavour.

INGREDIENTS

For the crust:

170 g (6 oz) almond flour

32 g (1 oz) keto powdered sugar

1 tsp cinnamon

6 tbsp butter, melted

For the filling:

720 g (1 lb 9 oz) cream cheese

130 g (4½ oz) keto powdered sugar

3 eggs

190 g (6¾ oz) unsweetened whole milk yoghurt

2 tsp lemon zest

1 tsp vanilla or almond extract

½ tsp salt

160 g (5½ oz) fresh or frozen raspberries, thawed if frozen

METHOD

Preheat oven to 150°C (300°F). Combine the almond flour, keto sugar, cinnamon and butter in a mixing bowl. Press into the bottom and sides of a 23-centimetre

(9-inch) springform pan. Bake for 12 minutes until beginning to brown.

While the crust is baking, combine the cream cheese and keto sugar in a stand mixer or a bowl with a hand mixer. Beat at medium speed until creamy (about 1 minute). Add the eggs individually, then add the yoghurt, lemon zest, extract and salt and blend thoroughly. Add the raspberries and fold in lightly at low speed.

Pour the mixture on top of the crust and use a knife to create a swirl design with the raspberries and batter.

Increase the oven temperature to 180°C (350°F). Place the springform pan in a baking tray and pour hot water into the tray until it's about halfway up the sides of the cheesecake.

Bake for 70–90 minutes until it is firm and set at the sides, but still jiggles in the centre when shaken. Remove from the water bath and cool.

Once cooled, remove from the pan, refrigerate for at least 6 hours, then serve chilled.

Wrap leftovers in plastic wrap, refrigerate for up to four days, or place in a Ziploc bag and freeze for up to two months. Thaw at room temperature for 1 hour or in the fridge overnight.

KETO CHOCOLATE MOUSSE

SERVES EIGHT

You'll never believe this super
simple, super creamy chocolate
mousse is low carb and low sugar
– but it is! Use raw cacao powder
for extra antioxidants and a rich
flavour, or traditional cocoa powder
for a more familiar-tasting treat.

INGREDIENTS

720 ml (24 fl oz) double cream

88 g (3 oz) powdered keto sweetener

88 g (3 oz) unsweetened raw cacao powder
or regular cocoa powder

2 tsp vanilla extract

1 tsp cinnamon

¼ tsp salt

Optional additions:

160 g (5½ oz) assorted berries

4 tbsp shredded coconut

4 tbsp sliced almonds

METHOD

In a large bowl, beat the cream at high speed with an electric hand mixer until it begins to thicken. Add the keto sweetener, cacao powder, vanilla extra, cinnamon and salt and beat at medium-high speed just until thick peaks form. Divide into eight individual bowls/cups or pour the mixture into one large serving bowl.

Chill for an hour, then serve with fresh berries, shredded coconut and almonds if desired.

Cover leftovers and refrigerate for up to three days.

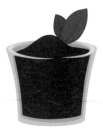

VEGAN KETO COCONUT PARFAITS

SERVES EIGHT (VEGAN)

With layers of coconut pudding, coconut whipped cream, berries and shredded coconut, this vegan parfait is perfect for a warm summer evening. You'll feel like you're on a tropical beach vacation as you enjoy this dessert!

INGREDIENTS

414 ml (14 fl oz) canned full-fat, unsweetened coconut milk

115 g (4 oz) granulated keto sweetener

½ tsp psyllium husk powder (available in most health stores)

1 tsp coconut or almond extract, or ½ tsp each

414 ml (14 fl oz) canned unsweetened coconut cream, refrigerated

33 g (1 oz) powdered keto sweetener

320 g (11¼ oz) raspberries, blueberries or sliced strawberries

50 g (2 oz) unsweetened shredded coconut

METHOD

Combine the coconut milk, granulated keto sugar and psyllium husk in a saucepan and cook over a medium heat, whisking until thick and bubbly. Remove from the heat, add the coconut or almond extract, place in a glass bowl and let sit for 5 minutes. Cover with cling film, making sure it is directly touching the pudding to prevent a film from forming, and refrigerate for 2 hours.

Remove from the fridge, beat with an electric hand mixer at medium-high speed until thick and creamy, and refrigerate an additional half hour.

In a separate bowl, place the coconut cream and powdered keto sweetener and beat with a hand mixer until thick.

In eight parfait glasses, layer one large spoonful each of coconut pudding and coconut whipped cream, followed by a sprinkling of berries and shredded coconut. Continue making layers until glasses are full, about three layers per parfait. Serve immediately or refrigerate until ready to serve. Cover leftovers and store in the fridge for up to three days.

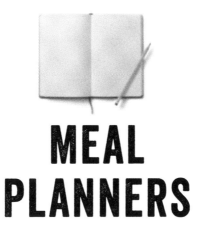

MEAL PLANNERS

IN THIS CHAPTER, YOU'LL FIND A TWO-WEEK MEAL PLANNER TO HELP YOU GET STARTED ON YOUR KETO JOURNEY. FEEL FREE TO SUBSTITUTE OTHER KETO-FRIENDLY INGREDIENTS AND MIX AND MATCH MEALS FROM DIFFERENT DAYS – CREATE A PLAN YOU WILL ENJOY AND STICK WITH!

BECAUSE DAILY CALORIE NEEDS WILL VARY BASED ON YOUR METABOLISM AND ACTIVITY LEVEL, PORTION SIZES AREN'T SPECIFIED. ADJUST PORTIONS AND ADD OR REMOVE SNACKS AS NECESSARY TO KEEP WITHIN YOUR IDEAL CALORIE COUNT.

WEEK ONE

	Monday	Tuesday	Wednesday
Breakfast	Eggs scrambled or fried in butter, served with sliced tomatoes	Bacon or turkey bacon, sliced avocado and tomatoes drizzled with olive oil	All-Purpose Keto Smoothie (p.45) made with strawberries, spinach, hemp and chia seeds
Lunch	Salad with greens, chicken breast, peppers and avocado, drizzled with olive oil and vinegar	Cabbage Crust Pizzas (p.50) or pizza made with store-bought keto crust, tomato sauce, grated cheese and veggie toppings	Avocado and Egg Salad (p.56) served with sliced cheese and turkey lunch meat, layered and rolled up
Dinner	Crispy and Creamy Parmesan Salmon (p.79) or any other low-carb salmon dish Steamed asparagus	Sautéed chicken thighs cooked in olive oil, skins on Steamed broccoli and cheese sauce	Baked ham served with Broccoli Rice (p.88)
Dessert/ snacks	Keto Fat Bomb (p.105) Store-bought keto ice cream	Handful of nuts of choice Keto Chocolate Mousse (p.111)	Pumpkin seeds Berries with dollop of Keto Chocolate Mousse (p.111)

	Thursday	Friday	Saturday	Sunday
Breakfast	Eggs with Kale, Mushrooms and Tomato (p.33)	Keto Berry Porridge (p.39)	Eggs scrambled with mushrooms in butter or olive oil	Keto Pumpkin Pancakes (p.36)
Lunch	Avocado, turkey breast, cheese and tomato served in a lettuce wrap or store-bought keto wrap Keto "coleslaw" (shredded cabbage, mayonnaise and vinegar)	Burger in a lettuce "bun" with tomato, avocado and keto "coleslaw" (shredded cabbage, mayonnaise and vinegar)	Baked or canned tuna with olives and tomatoes on mixed greens	Lettuce wrap with Hemp and Herb Pesto (p.82), cheese and sliced tomatoes
Dinner	Baked tofu with Broccoli Rice (p.88) or any veggies cooked in butter or olive oil	Courgette "Spaghetti" with Hemp and Herb Pesto (p.82) and Cheesy Keto Flatbread (p.94)	Steamed Broccoli with Hemp and Herb Pesto (p.82) and baked tofu or chicken, skins on	Meatballs with store-bought, keto-friendly marinara sauce and greens sautéed in olive oil
Dessert/ snacks	Keto Fat Bomb (p.105) Berries topped with shredded coconut	Celery sticks with nut butter Store-bought keto ice cream	Keto fat bomb (p. 105) Keto Raspberry-Lemon Cheesecake (p.108)	String cheese Keto Cheesecake (p.108)

WEEK TWO

	Monday	Tuesday	Wednesday
Breakfast	Cheese and green pepper omelette with salsa	Keto Berry Porridge (p.39)	Bacon or turkey bacon with avocado and salsa
Lunch	Grilled salmon with mixed greens, olive oil and vinegar dressing	Lettuce Wraps with Turkey and Avocado Dip (p.99) served with cherry tomatoes	Chicken salad served on a bed of greens with olives and tomatoes
Dinner	Pork Chops with Mushrooms (p.76) and sliced tomatoes	Courgette noodles with store-bought, keto marinara sauce prepared with ground beef Cheesy Keto Flatbread (p.94)	Eggs baked in a frying pan with Bolognese sauce Steamed cauliflower
Dessert/ snacks	Cucumbers with Avocado Dip (p.99) Berries with sugar-free chocolate chips	Handful of nuts of choice Full-fat unsweetened yoghurt with sugar-free chocolate chips	Keto Fat Bomb (p.105) Vegan Keto Coconut Parfaits (p.114)

	Thursday	Friday	Saturday	Sunday
Breakfast	All-Purpose Keto Smoothie (p.45) made with blueberries, kale and shredded coconut	Eggs fried in butter or olive oil served with sliced tomatoes and avocado	Berries topped with almond butter and shredded coconut	Pepper stuffed with scrambled eggs
Lunch	Salad with cubed baked tofu, greens, mushroom, olives, sliced almonds and olive oil vinaigrette	Grilled chicken atop mixed greens, served with Keto Cheesy Flatbread (p.94) or store-bought keto flatbread	Bacon Lettuce Tomato Wraps (p.53) with celery sticks	Salad made with chopped ham, mushrooms, tomatoes and mixed greens, with olive oil and vinegar
Dinner	Keto Butter Chicken (p.73) served with sauteed peppers	Baked salmon and asparagus roasted in olive oil	Keto Beef and Broccoli Stir-Fry (p.70)	Baked tofu Roasted Green Beans with Cherry Tomatoes and Almonds (p.91)
Dessert/ snacks	Celery sticks with sunflower seed butter Store-bought keto ice cream	Keto Fat Bomb (p.105) Full-fat unsweetened yoghurt with shredded coconut	Sunflower seeds Store-bought keto ice cream with shredded coconut	Almond butter with sugar-free chocolate chips Berries with shredded coconut

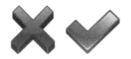

THE DOs
AND DON'Ts
OF KETO

ADOPTING A KETO DIET MAY FEEL OVERWHELMING, BUT BY KEEPING A FEW SIMPLE DOs AND DON'Ts IN MIND, YOU CAN EASILY STAY ON THE RIGHT TRACK AND EVEN ENJOY THE PROCESS. READ ON FOR SOME TOP TIPS FOR STAYING IN KETOSIS AND REMAINING HEALTHY ALONG THE WAY.

THE DOs:

1. DO talk to your doctor to ensure keto is safe for you.
2. DO plan meals to include the right balance of macronutrients.
3. DO prioritize heart-healthy fats, such as olive oil.
4. DO eat plenty of leafy greens.
5. DO enjoy low-sugar berries if you're craving sweets.
6. DO try new recipes and consume a variety of foods.
7. DO use keto strips or meters to test whether your body has entered ketosis.
8. DO remove non-keto foods from your kitchen if possible.
9. DO bring keto-friendly snacks with you outside the home.
10. DO remember to have fun and enjoy your healthy lifestyle!

THE DON'Ts:

1. DON'T consume more than 10 per cent daily calories from carbohydrates.
2. DON'T eat grains, starchy vegetables or high-sugar fruits.
3. DON'T overuse saturated and unhealthy fats.
4. DON'T consume sugar or artificial sweeteners.
5. DON'T forget to stay hydrated.
6. DON'T rely on the same few foods for every meal.
7. DON'T overeat just because a food is keto-approved.
8. DON'T expect physical changes to occur overnight.
9. DON'T forget to listen to your body and contact your doctor with any concerns.
10. DON'T give up. Sticking to a new diet is challenging, but the rewards make it worthwhile!

CONCLUSION

Now that you've reached the end of this book, you know much more about how keto works, how this diet can positively impact health and how to go about planning and following a keto meal plan. Whether you eat keto for a few weeks or a few months, you're well on your way to improving your health and well-being with all the benefits of the keto diet.

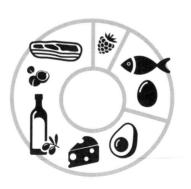

Have you enjoyed this book? If so, find us on Facebook at **Summersdale Publishers**, on Twitter at **@Summersdale** and on Instagram at **@summersdalebooks** and get in touch. We'd love to hear from you!

www.summersdale.com

IMAGE CREDITS